I0791424

Never **FORGET** to
REMEMBER
(My Journey Home)

Never **FORGET** to
REMEMBER
(My Journey Home)

By Robin Hunter

Title: **Never FORGET to REMEMBER, My Journey Home**

Author: Robin Hunter

Publisher: Robin Hunter, in association with Kindle Direct Publishing

Cover Design Layout: Robin Hunter

Art: Interior/Exterior:Robin Hunter

Interior Design Layout:Robin Hunter

ISBN: 9798512334126

Copyright©2021

Trademark™2021

Language: English

Printing and Binding: Amazon, Kindle Direct Publishing

Printed in the United States

MY MOMMY

Oh to be a mother. When I first could remember who you were it just made my heart very happy. I watched you maneuver through life as a mom, creating a new home for us children and all the while working two jobs. You appeared to be invincible. You made wanting to be a mom look so easy and effortless. Every important holiday, and birthday were always more than special. Telling the stories of your childhood and going to your family's church on Sunday and then going to your grandparent's house everyday after school was everything. Your mom, you and your sister lived five minutes down the road from your grandparent's house. The stories you would tell about your grandparents and their **"BIG WHITE HOUSE"**and how your school only had one room that still stands today. When I first saw your childhood school I thought this is it.The school is now more than 100 years old and is about 300 feet in front of your grandparent's house across the road. All those stories became my reality in 1974, when I had the wonderful opportunity to move from New York to Virginia as a child. I began to make my own memories in the **"BIG WHITE HOUSE"**, that is in front of the family's cemetery. I believe you forgot to mention to me there was a cemetery before I moved to Virginia. The cemetery became a quiet place for me to play and visit. I was never afraid.

This book is dedicated to my mommy **Charlotte Henrietta Grady-Pough**. Thank you mommy for taking your time with me and sharing your intimate stories. You were my first love and the main reason why I too wanted to become a mom. Now that you are no longer physically here with me, I pray that I am a reflection of what you wanted as a child. I never liked my name growing up but, it wasn't until God spoke to me and said she named you Robin because, just like a bird you should never be caged but, **"FREE"**

"FREE to BE ME"

For I am **"Charlotte's** daughter that was gifted to her by God to fulfill her purpose in this place.

"Never FORGET to REMEMBER"

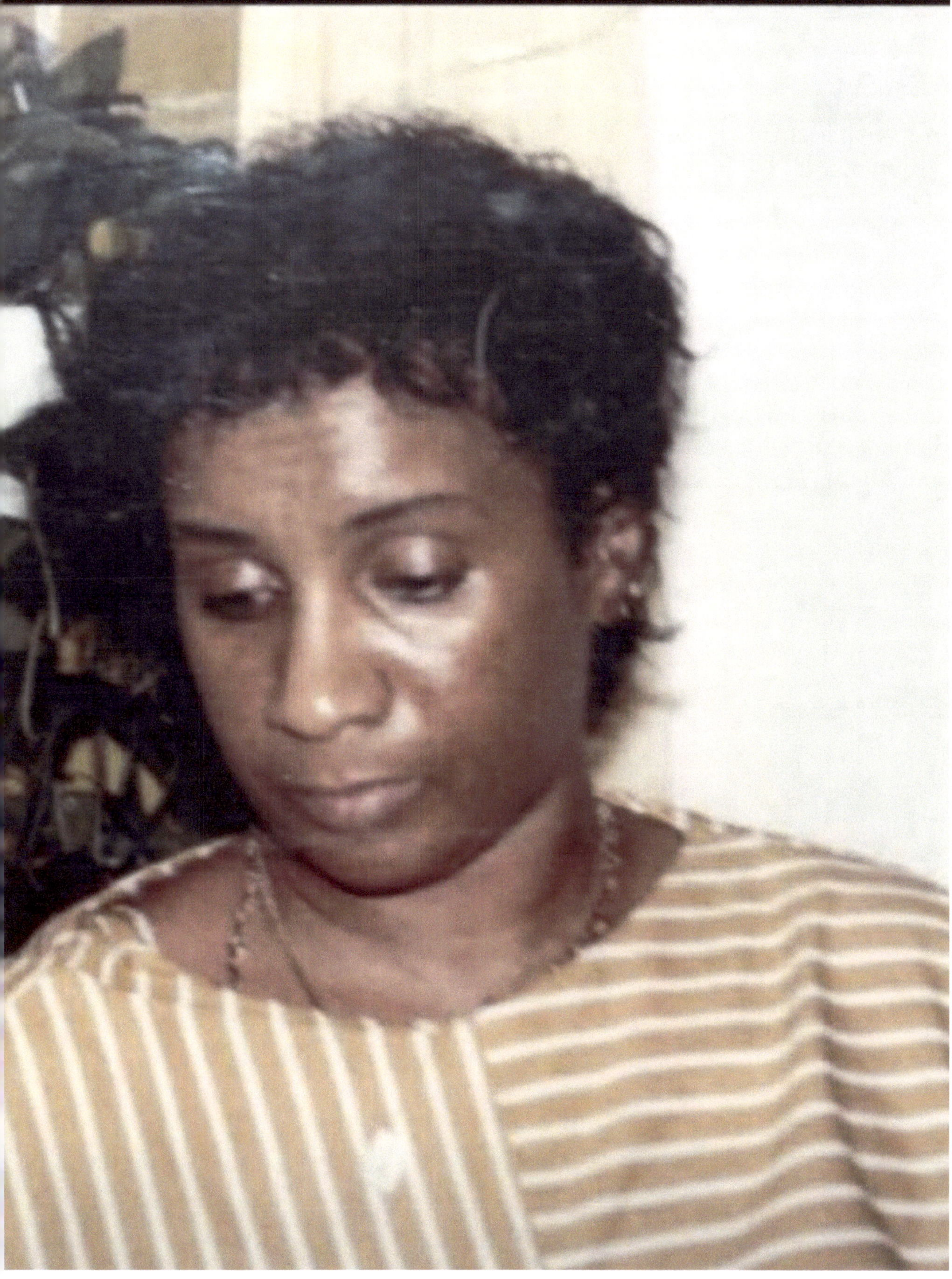

FOUR THE HARD WAY

We've all heard of **"three peas in a pod"**, well what about **"four the hard way"**
Meaning: The most difficult method or path. This term comes from the game of
craps, where it means making two dice come up with a pair of equal numbers
totaling the point.

Each individual had their very own unique style and meaningful place in each
other's life. On this day I was standing behind the camera to capture this frozen
moment in time as if it were yesterday. Although I can't remember what made
them want to take this picture that day, now I'm glad they did. In the words of Ice
Cube **"today was a good day"**. I am wherever she is.
**From left to right: Wawa, Momma (Blanche Lucille Johnson), Walter Davis
and Mommy**

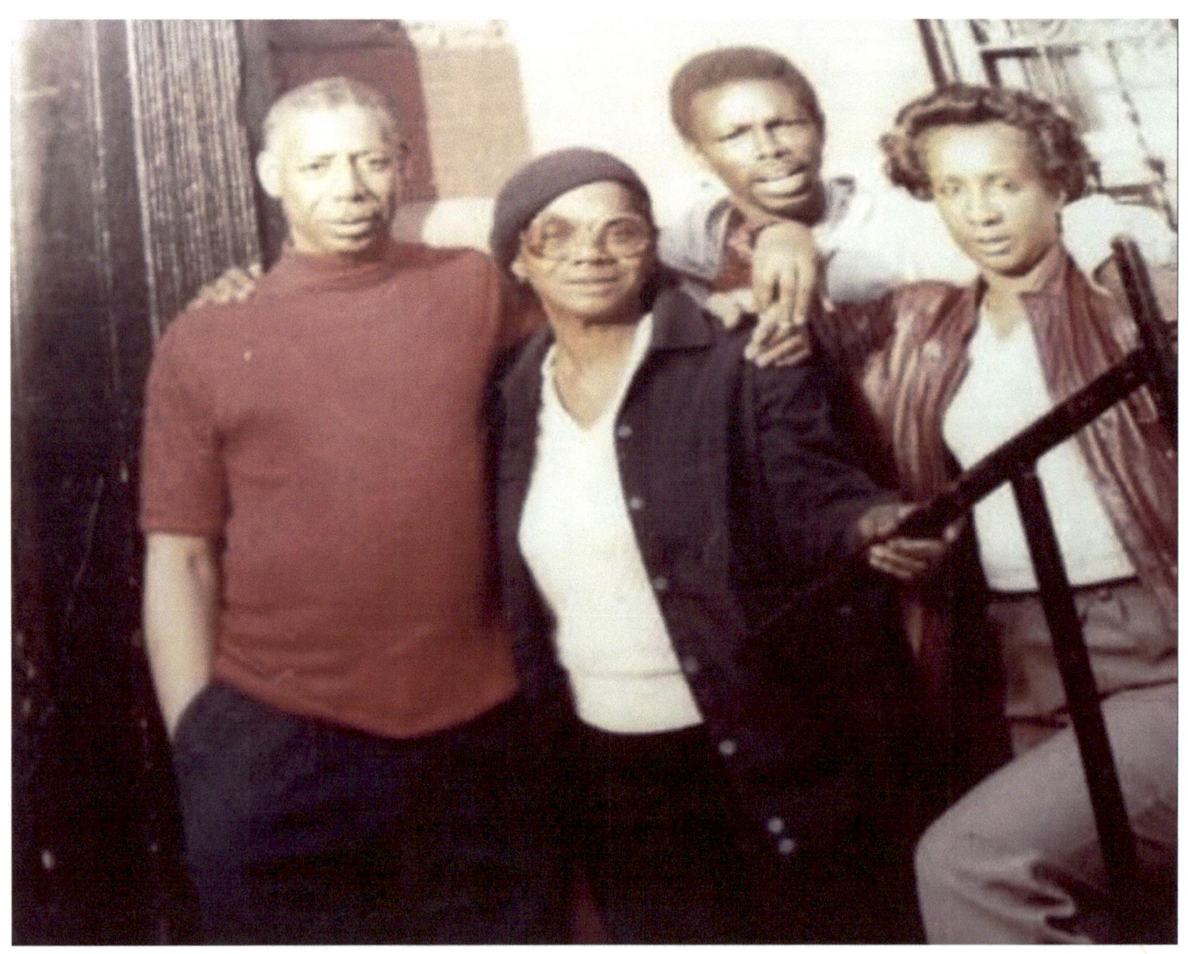

"THE BIG WHITE HOUSE"
CHARLOTTE and FLORENCE GRANDPARENTS HOME

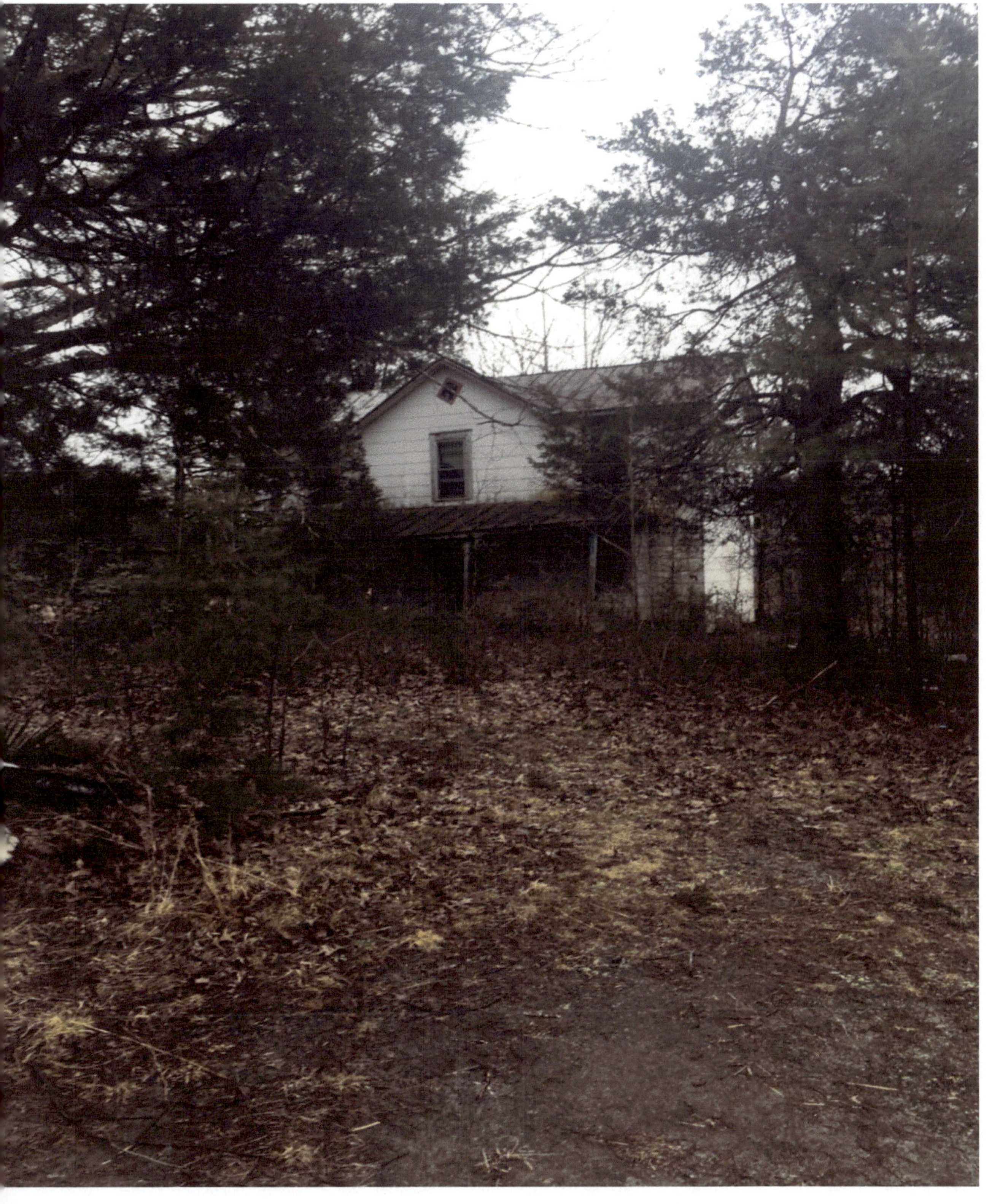

CHARLOTTE and FLORENCE CHILDHOOD HOME

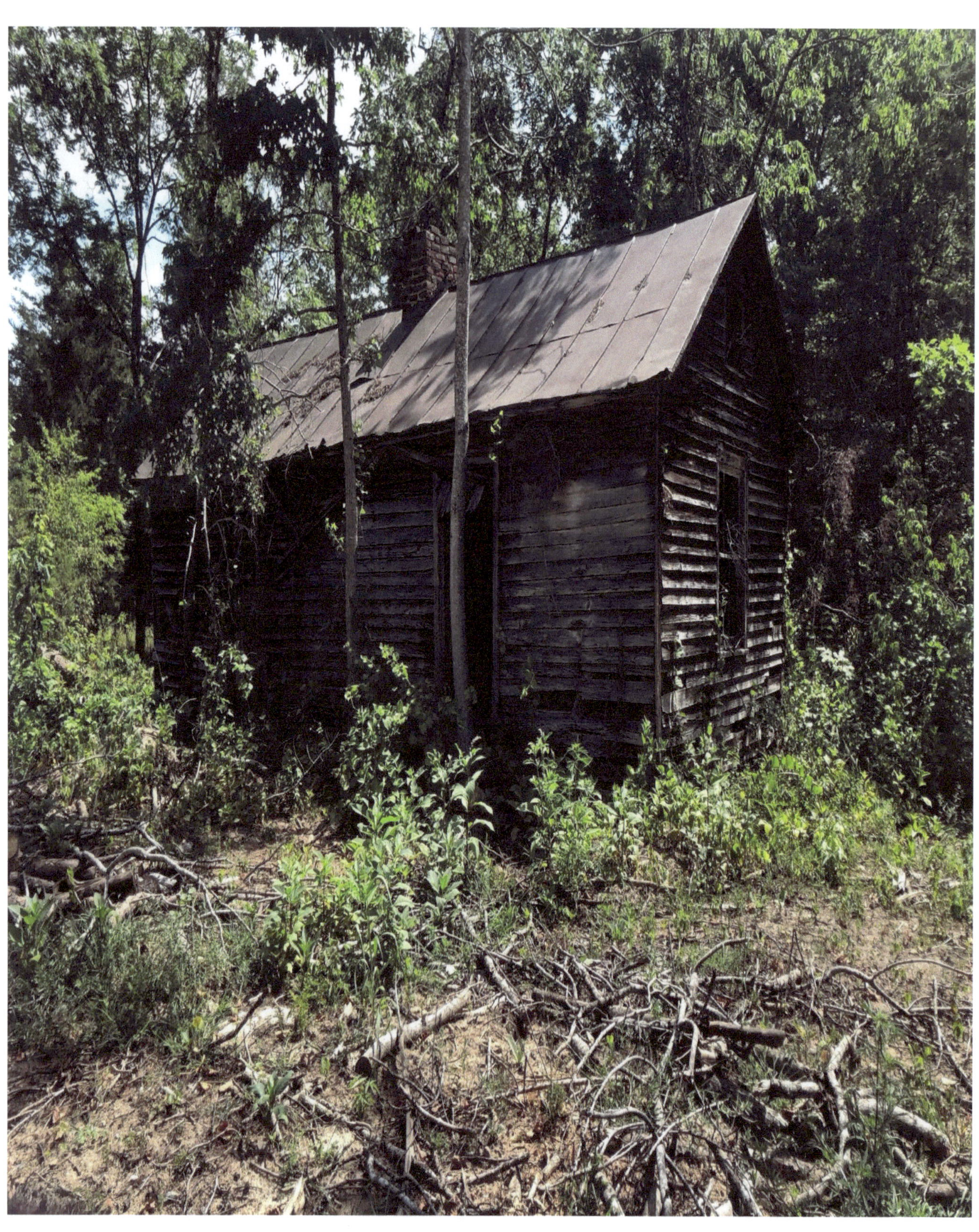

THE ONE ROOM SCHOOL : GRADES 1st-12th

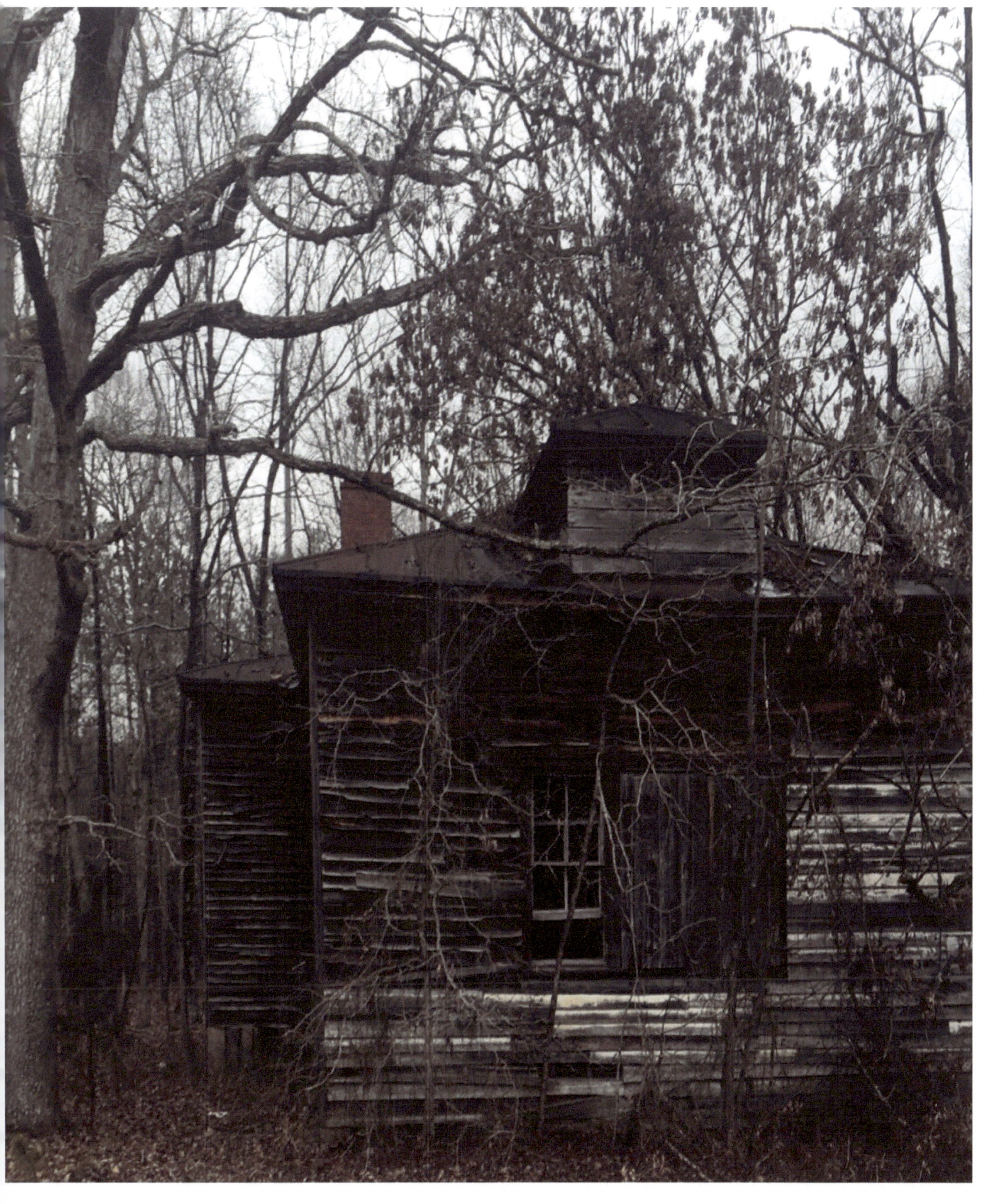

AUNT FLORENCE

My Aunt Florence and I had a very special relationship. My mom and aunt Florence could almost be mistaken for twins. Those two had an undeniable special bond as sisters. I remember her calling my name countless times when she came to visit me here in Virginia. I was always into something. I loved to make mud pies, running outside with no shoes and my favorite was messing with her. She would say "sputnik", that was the name my grandfather called me. "Come on I would say let's go play hide and seek". Her response was "sputnik I'm tired". She actually climbed one of our peach trees behind the house. I looked for her for at least fifteen minutes. I went to my mother crying saying I can't find her. My mother came outside and saw her in the tree and then said "Florence stop hiding from her". My aunt must have thought that sputnik is crazy and she told me to hide. I couldn't imagine why she would be tired in the first place. Earlier that day Mama, cousin Arthur and Aunt Florence and I went walking down the road to pick blackberries from the thorny bush on the side of the road. Mama also chopped the head off of one of our chickens to prepare for dinner. I do remember saying "I'm not eating that" and she said, "where do you think the chickens from the store come from"? I just looked and walked away as the kitchen smelled of that poor chicken being boiled in the pot. My aunt went to rest because she was tired. I must have forgotten that older people needed their rest. My aunt had to be about thirty five or thirty six years old, but to me that was old.

My morning routine when my Mama came to stay with us was to get up really early and we would eat peaches and ice cream for breakfast. My Mom came into the dining room and thought I made it for myself. Mom said "Robin who gave you those peaches and ice cream"? My response was "Mama". Mama was standing off in the kitchen and her response was priceless, "Charlotte that's just milk and fruit". My mother just shook her head and walked away. My times when my aunt and grandma came to visit were always memorable. I'll never forget to remember. Pictures may fade but the memories last forever.

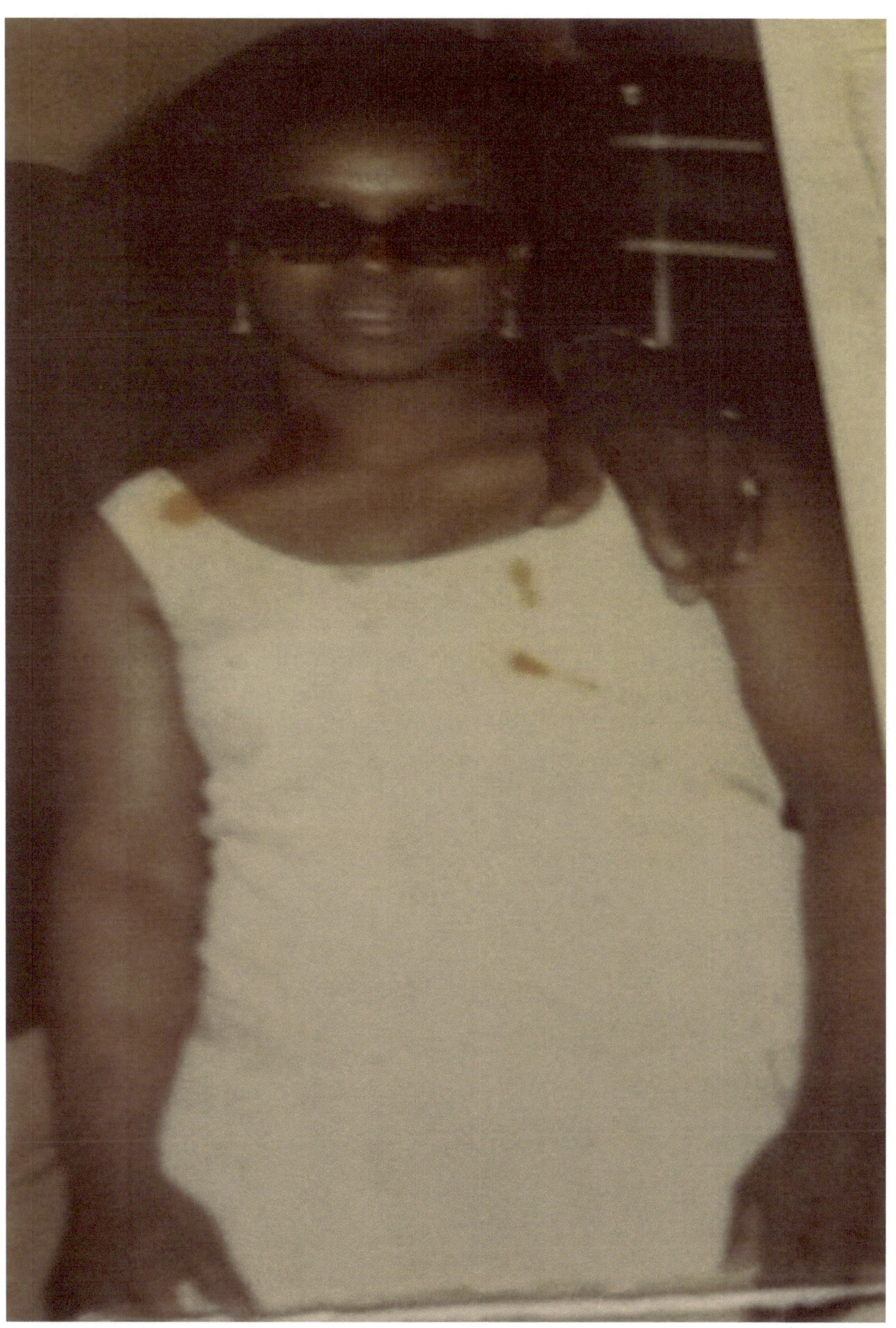

CHARLES HENRY BUCKNER
(MY GRANDADDY)

My GRANDADDY, what can I say? I don't know how many children got their first driving lesson on Interstate 95 at the age of four sitting on their grandfather's lap. I had no idea how much he loved me and wanted me to feel special. He appeared to let me drive with confidence, all the while he knew the car was on autopilot and he was controlling everything. Whenever my grandfather came to visit, it always felt like Christmas, not because of gifts, but it was how he was just as excited to see me as I was to see him. One Christmas did stand out for me, it was the Christmas I saved my money because I wanted to buy him a gold chain. I got my grandfather the gold chain and he thought it was the best gift ever. He couldn't wait to put the chain on. My grandfather died when I was twelve years old. I remember standing over top of his casket and looking at his neck, there was the gold chain peaking out at me. His wife leaned over and said "he never took the chain off". All I remember is that when I looked at the chain it looked "blueish green". As I got older I thought about the chain and I remember his wife saying "he never took it off". My grandfather was a very classy man, he had to have known that the chain wasn't real. He sported the chain in true elegance because it was a gift from his grand-daughter. I never got the chance to ask my grandfather, why did he name me "sputnik"? GRANDADDY I miss you every day, until we see each other again. Oh by the way my feet finally can touch the pedals.

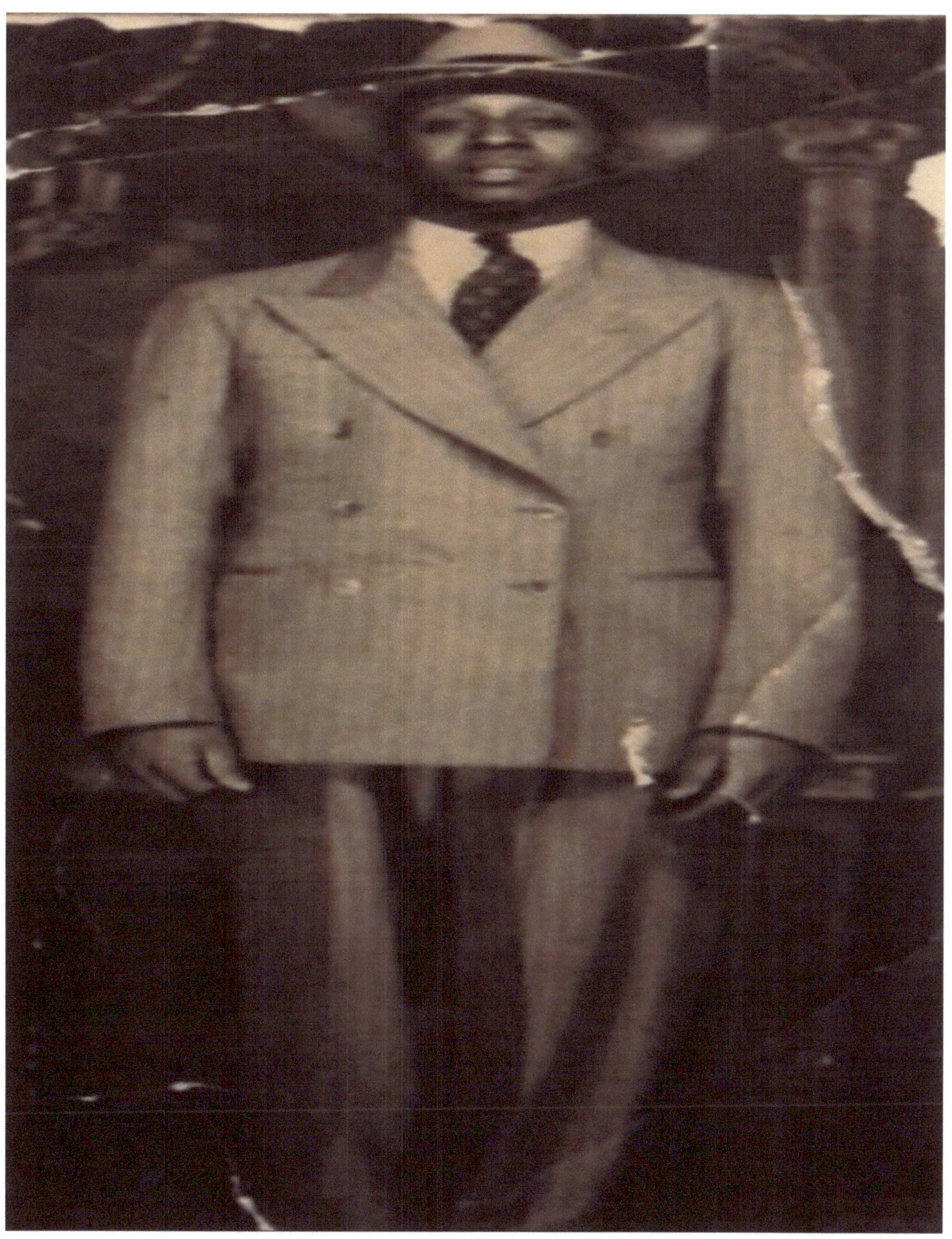

THE VILLAGE

The village includes many people that bring a variety of life's experience that enrich our very own lives. They bring their childhood stories of fun and laughter as well as pain. Each of those individuals we must understand had their very own village as well. When we take the time to sit still long enough to hear their stories, our hearts should become more compassionate. Some of these individuals have arrived with fragmented pieces of others attached to them. Then we have those who made it this far by barely hanging on. Once we find out that the village many of them came from, we can see how they just did the best they could with what they had to work with. We can't judge a person for utilizing the tools that they have readily available in their tool box.

FAMILY   **FRIENDS**   **AUNTS**

COUSINS   **UNCLES**

TEACHERS   **NEIGHBORS**   **GRANDPARENTS**

FRIENDS

Always remember that good friends along the way to your final destination can always be of some use (A good laugh, A shoulder to lean on, A teacher, A listener, An advisor and so much more). The intersection of roads allows us to make very valuable decisions on how to maneuver and help us grow. The creation of these human structural paths are sometimes smooth but, it's those rocky ones that make you feel uncomfortable and unsure. If we go our separate ways today, may we find our way back to each other stronger, better and have something of value to offer one another.

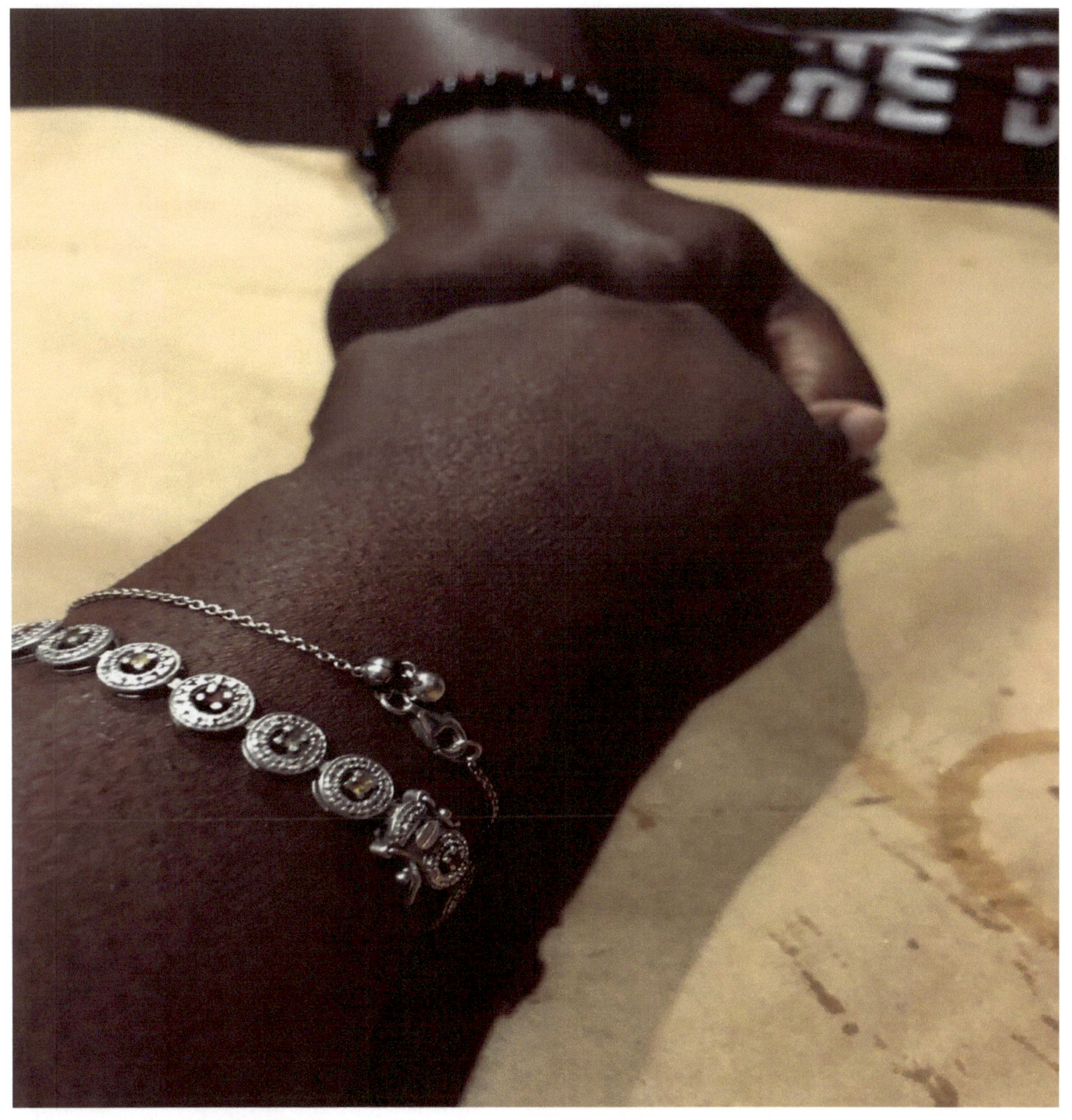

LAUREL HILL BAPTIST CHURCH
Est. 1868
(OUR FAMILY CHURCH)

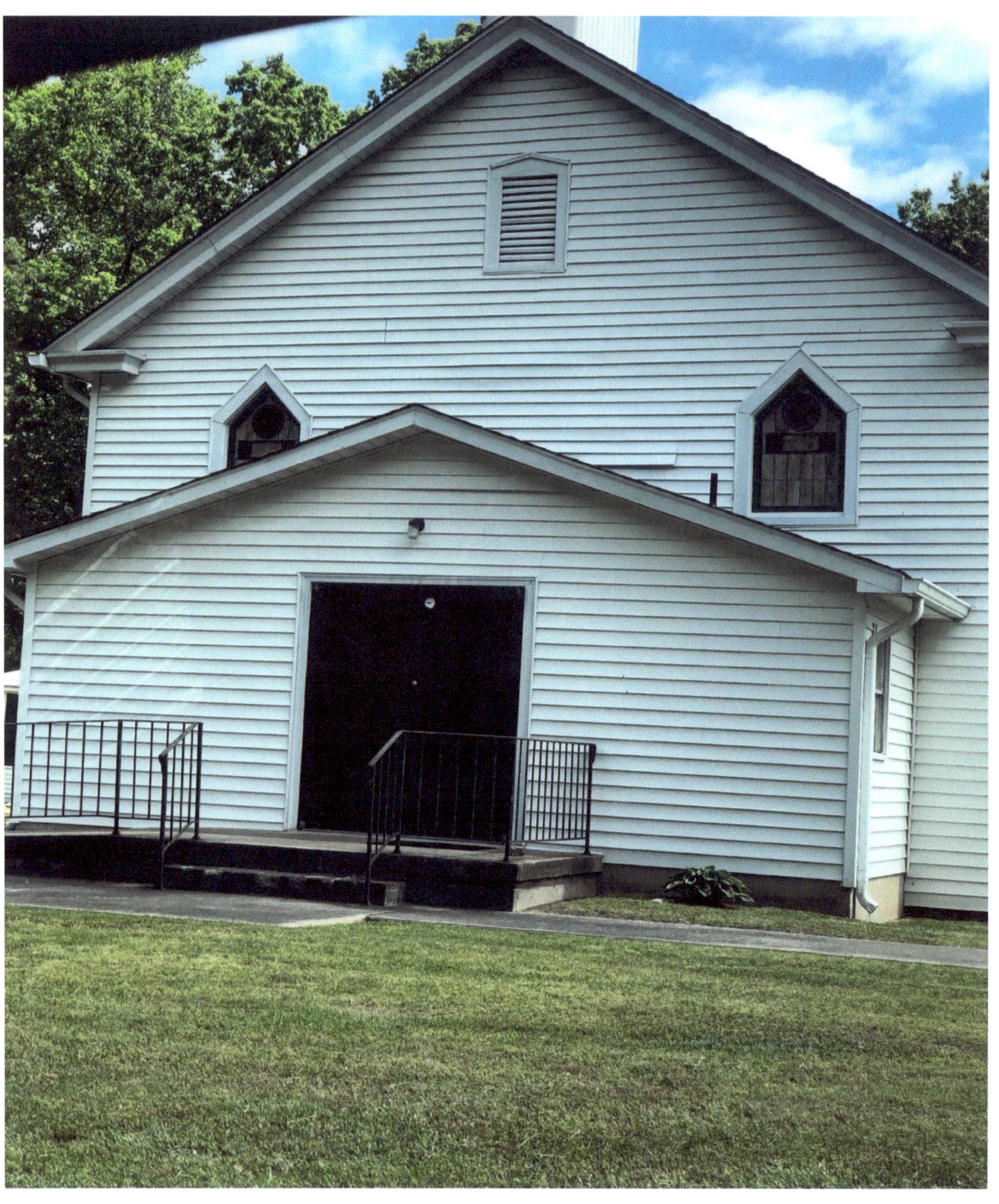

Sunday was sometimes the best day of the week for me because it felt like I was heading off to school. I was unable to attend primary school when I first moved to Virginia because of my age and late birthday. During the week my siblings had lessons to complete from school and household chores to be done at home, so Saturday mornings at home for them and myself was time spent watching "Soul Train " and cartoons. I made sure that my chores were done ahead of time. Saturday's seemed to go on forever and then before I knew it, it was Sunday morning and a car moving only about ten miles per hour was headed down the road to pick me up for **ALL DAY CHURCH**. The car was driven by one of my mother's elderly cousins, her name was cousin Mildred Coles. Her home was three houses down the road within walking distance from ours. We would visit her house as children on Saturday because her side entrance was set up as a little candy store. Her home always smelled like oatmeal cookies. Sunday church felt just like I imagined school was for my sisters. We had all day lessons from morning to afternoon and then we were the last ones to leave because we had to help clean for the following week. I enjoyed church as a child especially in the summer because the ice cream truck and candy man came. When I returned home in the late afternoon from church, I would have to discuss what I learned in church and recite a prayer before bedtime. I was baptized at nine years old in 1978 and I remember that day as being a huge celebratory event. Every year since my baptism the church still has a family Bible Convocation every third Sunday in August. A small church with a huge impact on people from years past to present. These are a few moments and memories that helped to shape a child's spiritual journey.

MINERAL, VIRGINIA
(MY PLACE OUT OF NO PLACE)

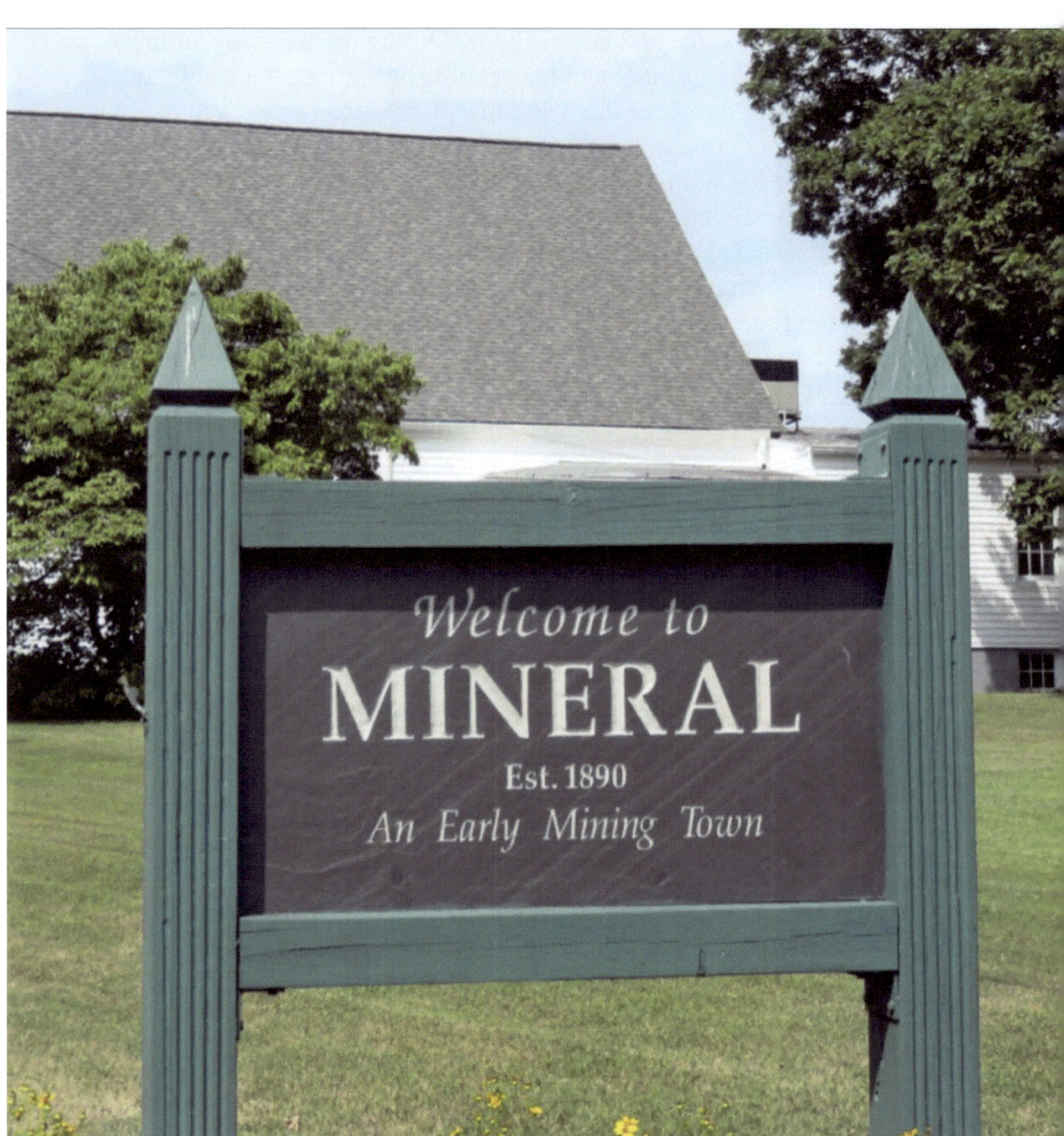

Mineral, Virginia was established in 1890. The purpose of this little town was to mine. Workers would come to work and retreat back home. Somehow it made more sense to set up a homestead instead of retreating home daily. According to the 2019 census, the town of Mineral population was estimated at 523 residents. I remember moving to this quiet small place in 1974, when I was four years old turning five. I cried for at least a week to go back home to New York, only to be told by my mother this is your home. This was such sad news at first. As years passed, I began to understand why my mother loved this place so much. At first glance, there's just dirt roads, trees for miles, and just strange sounds all day long and it got dark way too early. Did I mention there's only one street light that didn't cascade very far. My new home was my great grandparents' home that was in front of our family's cemetery. As a little girl my mind was very creative. Ironically for me instead of being afraid of the cemetery, I would go to visit often. What may appear to be a frightening place for many children, I found it to be my very own place of peace.

Mineral is a very small town located in Louisa County. This town would've never been heard of if it had not been for the 2011 earthquake of 5.8 magnitude that originated here. The earthquake lasted less than one minute and it was felt from Florida all the way to Canada. This town made history and is still talked about to this day. The surrounding counties within 35 miles of the earthquake were impacted greatly for several years after. Areas such as Louisa, Goochland, Bumpass, Cuckoo, Spotsylvania and Trevillian had millions of dollars in damage. The schools in Louisa had to close because their educational symbolic structure that stood for seventy three years was completely destroyed.

LOUISA COUNTY HIGH SCHOOL
1938-2011
(original structure destroyed in earthquake)

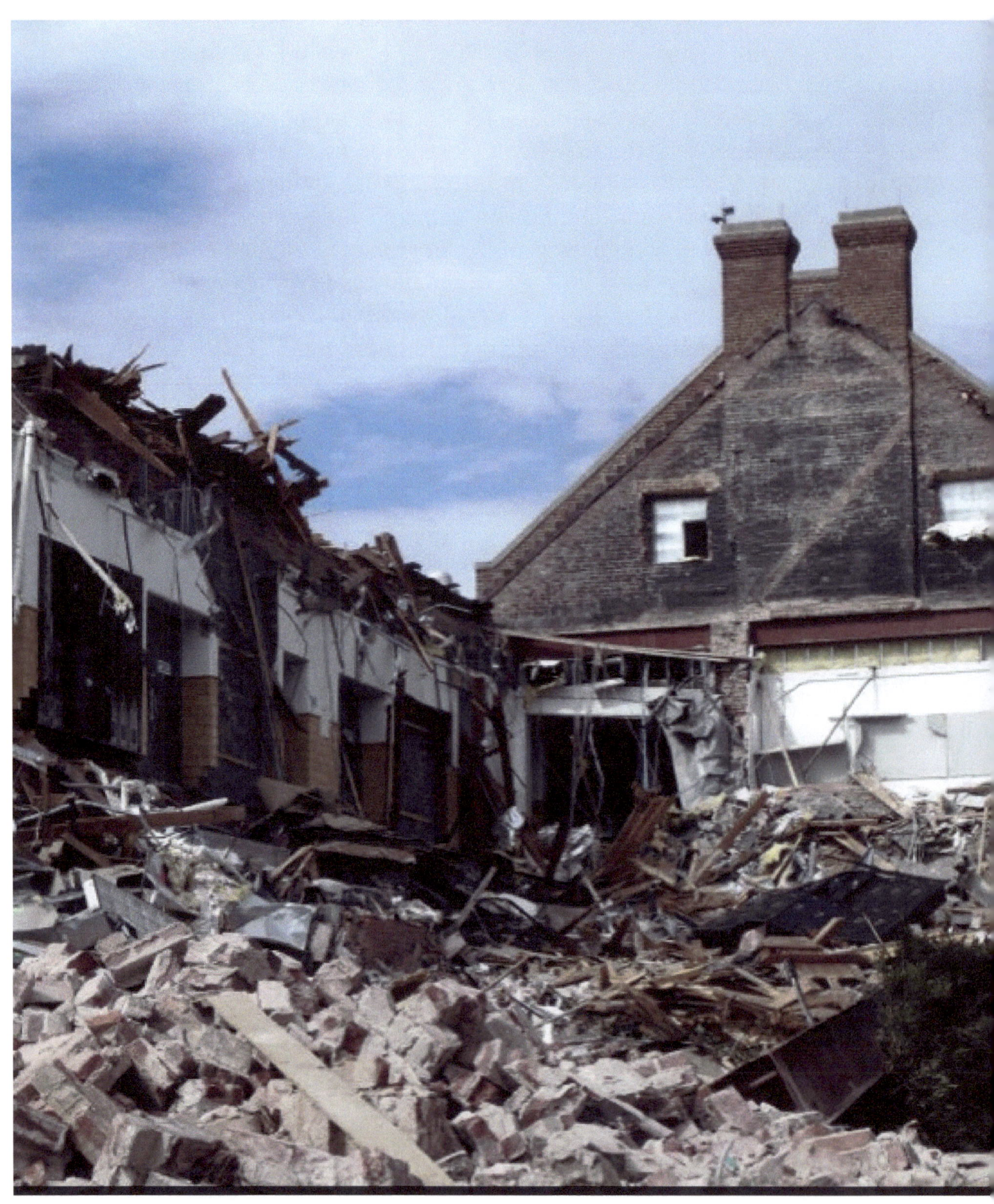

MINERAL TRAIN DEPOT
(first built in 1851 and then reconstructed in 1880)

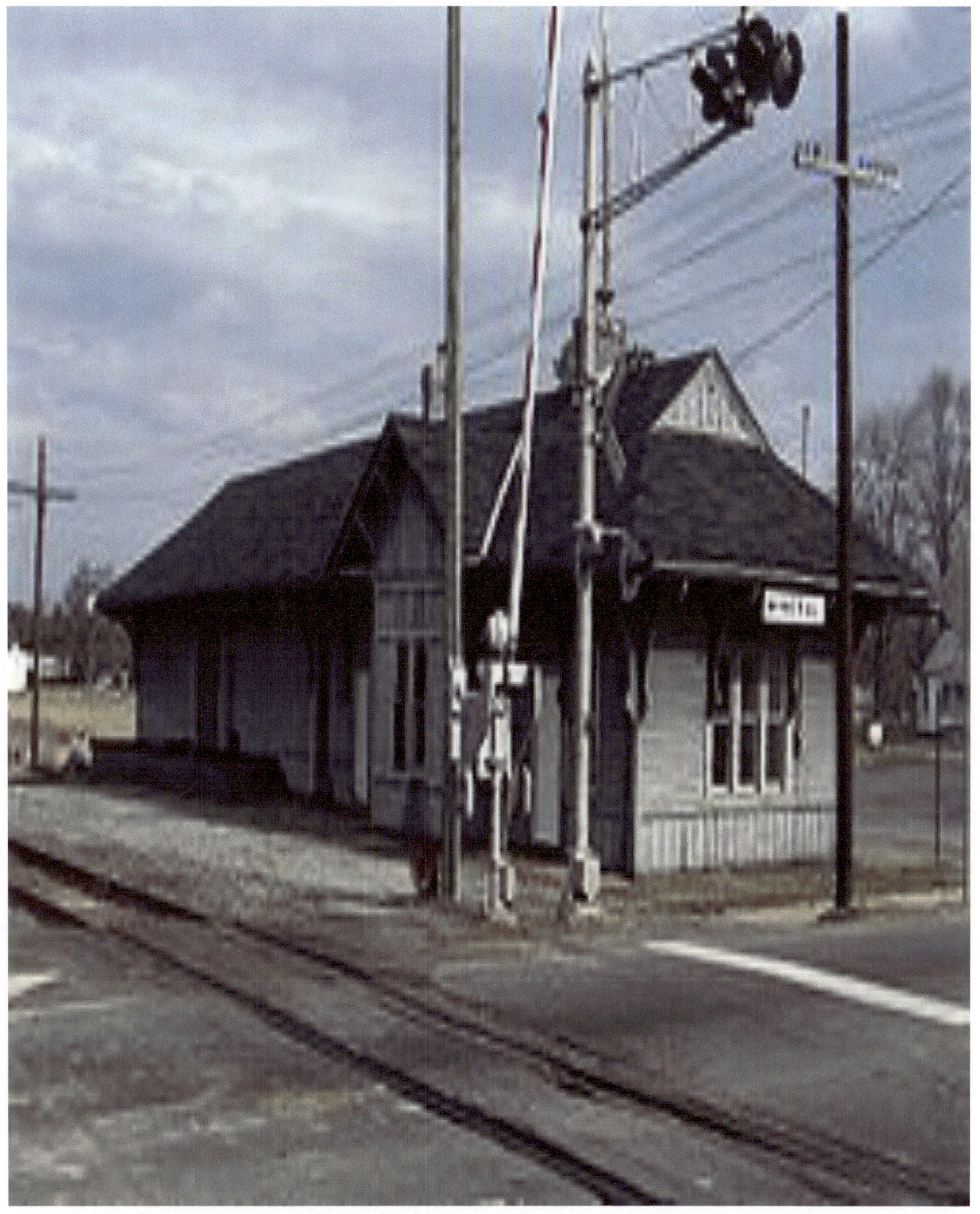

MADELINE NEWSON
(MY MOTHER -IN LAW)

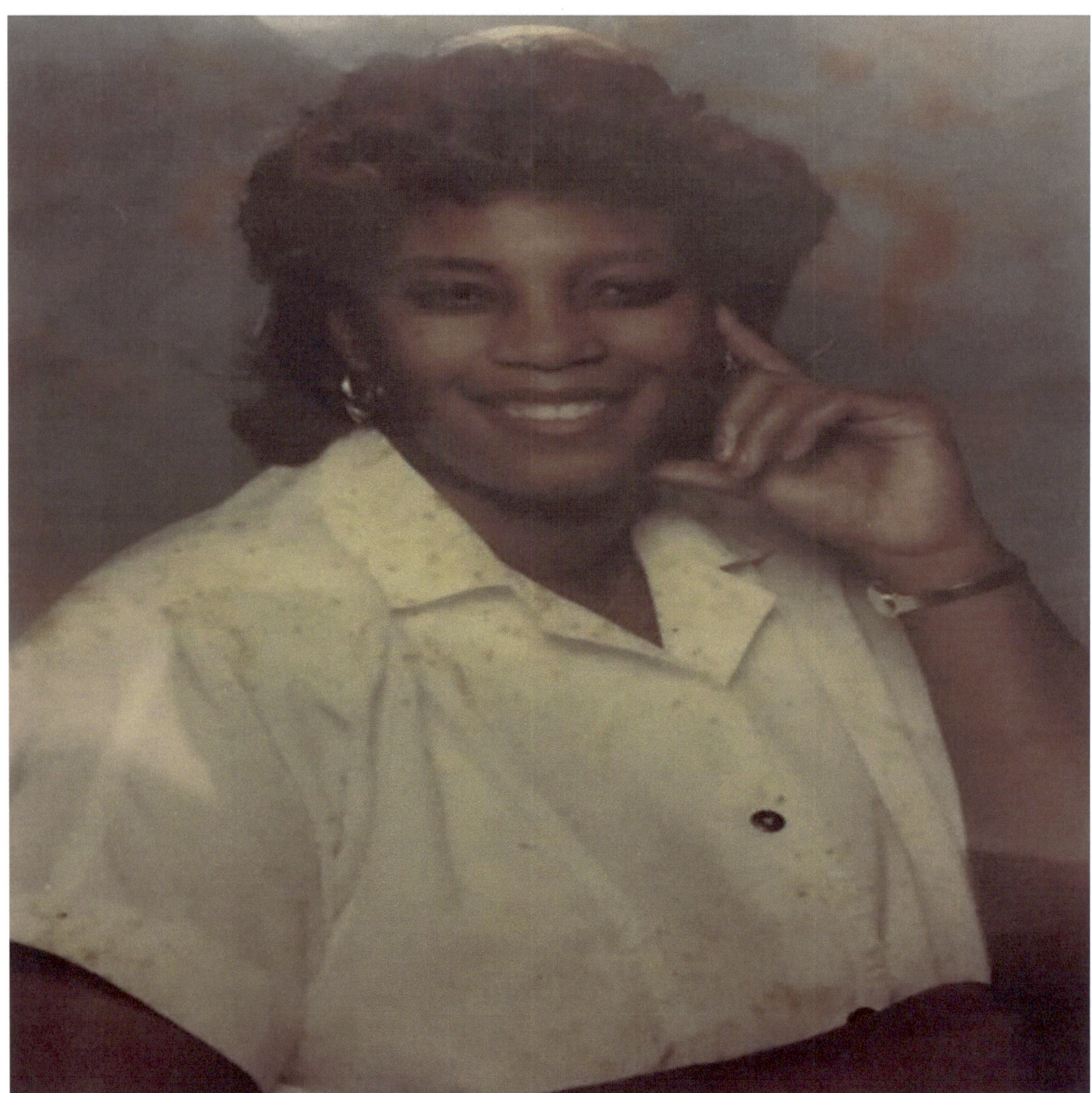

Never FORGET to REMEMBER, the people you encounter that have made
sacrifices that have unknowingly changed your life. Sometimes people give so
much to others that they forget to save just a little for themselves. Never FORGET
to REMEMBER, that when it's your heart's desire to do something, GOD WILL
HONOR THAT. Never FORGET to REMEMBER, to whom much is given so
much more is required. Grandma Madeline we all miss you and love you.

**I'll
NEVER
FORGET
TO
REMEMBER**

(LOVE ALWAYS ME)